# Natural Acne Treatments

## The Best Homemade Remedies
## For Acne Damaged Skin

ALISON BARNES

# DEDICATION

This book is dedicated to all those who suffer with the embarrassment of acne and skin related problems.

Know that there is help and natural solutions available.

# A QUICK START: AN OLD ENGLISH REMEDY

*There is an old English remedy for flushing toxins out of your body that is centuries old and easy to do.*

*It involves diluting a teaspoon or two of Organic Apple Cider Vinegar in a glass of water and drinking this three times a day. Organic is preferred as it is unprocessed and retains more of the original beneficial minerals. Diluting the Organic Apple Cider Vinegar helps minimize damage to tooth enamel.*

*Organic Apple Cider Vinegar helps to flush out toxins from the liver and intestinal tract and enables these systems to work more efficiently.*

*This is a very good tip on clearing and preventing acne because it causes cleansing from the inside out. This simple tip will work wonders. Just try it for 1 month in combination with a good skin cleaning regime and you will see dramatic results.*

*Just add one teaspoon of Organic Apple Cider Vinegar to a bottle or glass of water that you drink and do this three times each day.*

# Table of Contents

# Welcome

Welcome to the "wonderful" world of acne.

Thank you for purchasing this book, and don't worry. Your acne solution is in here.

Most of us, even those of us who do not suffer from extreme acne, have dealt with acne at some point in our life. By the time you are done reading this acne book, you will have a much better understanding of what you are going through, what causes it, what you can do to help prevent and treat your acne, and you will also know that you are not alone.

It is best to read this acne book through all the way one time and then use the sections that you need for reference.

I have tried to include the most important sections toward the front of the acne book so that you can begin making productive skin changes early.

Best of luck, I hope this information helps you as it has helped me.

Alison

# What is Acne?

Acne is a term whose definition is used very broadly.

**Acne is basically plugged up skin pores that result in blackheads, whiteheads, pimples, cyst type pimples and big lumps.**

Acne is also the source of many years of depression for a lot of people and while it is most common in teen agers, anyone, regardless of their age can develop acne.

Acne does not discriminate, in addition to occurring on your face, it can also occur on your chest, your back, your shoulders and upper arms, and even your butt.

Severe acne can lead to permanent scarring and is extremely upsetting. It is not life threatening, but if you are thirteen and already feeling awkward and out of place, having acne can certainly feel life threatening.

If you are already an adult and develop acne for the first time, you may realize it is not life threatening, but it does not make you feel any better about it.

**Acne extends beyond physical damage and "scars" the self-image of the individual.**

# Types of Acne

There are different types of acne. The most common type is called a lesion.

Lesions can be external or internal. It is, by definition, a physical change in tissue caused by disease or injury. Lesions can be smaller like blackheads and whiteheads or they can be large like cysts.

Both sizes are difficult to deal with and just because blackheads are smaller, they can be just as damaging as the larger cyst type acne.

Within each type of acne, there are mini-types like blackheads and whiteheads.

Figuring out how to deal with acne is dependent upon what type of acne you have.

The first step is to see a dermatologist to determine what type of acne you are facing.

# What Causes Acne?

At this point, I'm sure you have a pretty good idea of what foods to avoid and what foods you should be eating. This is the easy part.

Knowing about foods and knowing that keeping your face clean can help prevent acne, you may be wondering what actually causes acne.

Is there one specific thing that is making you break out or are there a variety of causes that make you break out?

As previously discussed <u>the number one cause of acne is clogged pores and follicles</u>.

As a teenager, your hormones are raging and your skin hygiene is probably not the greatest. At this time, more than ever in your life, you should be hyper aware of what is going on in your body. If you know you break out after exercising, be diligent in the hot water, soap, cold water treatment. This alone will make a great improvement in the condition of your skin.

Dirt, dead skin cells, and makeup and sweat clog pores and follicles.

**There is no single cause for acne.**

It might be the food you eat. It could be stress. It could be your skin is not being kept clean enough. It could be just about anything. So treating acne can take some time. <u>There is no miracle first time cure because everyone's body is different</u>. Not eating dairy might clear up my skin, but it could be bad for yours.

**The best way is through trial and error until you can determine what is probably causing acne for you.**

It can be frustrating and disheartening to realize that there is no magic wand or magic pill to get rid of your acne. There are however, a lot of things you can do to help prevent and treat the acne you already have.

# What To Do About Acne

### Step 1: Blackhead Treatment

There are things you can do if you are afflicted with blackheads. Even if the blackheads aren't severe enough to be considered acne, they are still pesky and hard to get rid of.

Blackheads occur when follicles get blocked by dead skin and dirt. Although blackheads are on the surface of your skin, the problem is just underneath, which is why it is almost impossible to pop one. Blackheads show you where major pores are blocked and bacteria begin to grow.

**How to rid yourself of blackheads – wash your face properly.** Step one is to soak a washcloth in hot water, the hotter the better.

Apply the hot washcloth to the area where the blackheads are until it starts to cool off. This opens your pores.

Use soap (personal preference is Zest because it dries out my skin, but the choice is yours to make) or a skin scrub and scrub your face.

Rinse your face with lukewarm water and then

Rinse your face with ice water. The ice water closes your pores back up to prevent dirt and dead skin from getting back in.

This won't have an immediate effect; it will probably take a few days to a week for you to really notice the difference. Once you see the difference, keep doing it, fanatically. If you miss one time, get ready for an acne breakout.

Dirt and dead skin cells are something that cannot be avoided, so you have to keep washing your face this way. It sounds simple but you must follow this regime as often as you can each day.
**Makeup: The number one problem for female acne.**

Makeup is bad for your skin! You are putting "plugs" directly into your pores each time you apply makeup.

This is not to say that you *have* to stop wearing makeup (although I would). However, you will need to <u>wash your face before putting makeup on</u> - <u>with the cold water treatment last</u>, this helps to close up your pores and helps to prevent the makeup from getting in there.

It is even more important to wash off your makeup at night the same way. This gives your skin time to breathe without the extra dirt, skin cells, and makeup while you're sleeping.

## Step 2: Your Diet and Acne

Are you aware that the foods you eat can help prevent or encourage acne? Let's take at look at some foods that are not good for your skin.

It is a common held belief that <u>dairy products</u> are the cause of most acne. There is something in the pasteurization process of milk (all types except soy) yogurts, cream, and cheese that can lead to an allergic reaction that produces acne.

If you think this might be the cause of your acne, stop the intake of dairy products and supplement your calcium, vitamin D, and protein through other foods and vitamin supplements. This alone might clear you up.

<u>Caffeine</u> and <u>alcohol</u> can also be contributors as well as <u>spicy foods</u>. Each effects your heart rate by making it faster and increasing the amount of sweat you produce or by slowing it down (alcohol) and preventing the amount of sweat you release.

Exercise can have the same affect if you do not wash your acne infected area thoroughly afterwards.

Candy, chocolate, rice, refined flour, garlic, mushrooms, and oysters are also at the top of the list of foods that can produce acne. Like with pasteurized dairy products, acne can be the result of an allergic reaction to those foods.

> **Remember, the allergic reaction is not severe enough that you need medical attention, but produces acne instead.**

The good news about changing your eating patterns to try to figure out what might be causing acne is that **most of the food you are eliminating is food you shouldn't be eating on a regular basis anyway**.

Dairy has a lot going for it, but it also has a lot against it. The most obvious is how fatty dairy products tend to be. You may be okay drinking non-fat milk, but are you okay eating non-fat cheese?

**My** suggestion for switching your diet to see if that is aiding in your acne issues is to do a different thing each week. Start on a Monday and do not eat dairy products for an entire week. If your acne starts to clear up and nothing else has changed, that might be it. If dairy seems to have no affect, try a week without chocolate.

**Test and Retest: Do a different thing each week**. Experiment and remember that it may not be obvious, i.e., chocolate may contain milk products, so is it the milk products or the chocolate that is causing your problem? Try milk free chocolate, test and retest.

As you identify food or foods that cause your acne, **write them down and stop eating them**.

### Step 3: Foods that help clear up Acne

If you have gone through the process of eliminating foods that may cause acne and nothing has changed, you may be wondering if there are foods that help clear up acne. The short answer is, "No, but…"

No single food or combination of foods will clear up your acne. However, **eating a balanced diet will help because improving your overall health will help.**

**Eat a lot of fruits and vegetables**. In addition to vitamins, fruits and vegetables provide calcium and protein.

**Make sure you are not getting too much protein from red meat**. The average intake of protein depends on your weight in kilograms (or pounds). I weight 54kgs (137 lbs) so my protein intake should be 54 grams 0.14 lbs). The granola bars I eat for breakfast contain 21 grams (0.05 lbs) of protein (nuts and sunflower seeds!) so after breakfast, I have already taken in half of my protein for the day. 1kg = 1,000 grams = 2.54 lbs, if you need to do these conversions.

The reason it is important to not take in the majority of your protein through red meat, is because red meat is not really good for you. Burgers, steaks, tacos, whatever you eat that has meat in it, is probably going to be fatty (think cholesterol and clogged arteries).

Red meat elevates your bad cholesterol. Eat chicken, turkey, or a vegetarian based burger instead. We need protein for energy and to sweat and that helps clear the skin. Remember, protein is good, but protein from red meat is not so good.

**Drink a lot of water**. [This is my **NUMBER 1** personal acne prevention secret]. Most of us know that water flushes your system. It is not only important for headaches and hang-over's, but for the overall health of your skin and body.

**Water** helps flush the toxins out and, if you normally drink enough water, **you should double that amount to help flush your body faster and more efficiently**. This can help clear up your skin.

**I drink at least the equivalent of 10 eight ounce glasses of water each day.** It is the first thing I do in the morning and the last thing I do each night. At first this will seem like a lot, but you get used to it.

Each person is different, but **I believe that increasing my water consumption helped my skin more than any other change that I made.**

The best part about water is that it is easy and free! Be sure to read the next section on vitamins and supplements as too much water can dilute and flush these essentials from your system. If you drink a lot of water, you need to supplement with vitamins.

### Step 4: Back to the better diet thing...

If you are already eating well, and have cut down on fats and are getting plenty of fruits and vegetables you may want to **try nutritional supplements** in addition. Supplements can help decrease inflammation and infection. The reason is they *feed* **your skin**, and help prevent acne and repair tissue.

### Essential Skin Care Nutrients

Vitamin A

Vitamin B complex

Vitamin B2

Vitamin B6

Pantothenic acid

Vitamin C

Vitamin E

Vitamin F

Calcium

Potassium

# Multi-Vitamins and Minerals

**Multi-vitamins and minerals,** in addition to fruits and vegetables, can give your body the boost it needs to help fight off acne. Keep in mind that your body prefers a fresh intake of vitamins each day, but most of us do not get the daily vitamins, minerals, and proteins that we need.

**A** supplement can be a great way to help. If the supplement means you have a little too much of one vitamin or another, our bodies are made in such a way to flush out what we don't need of water soluble vitamins.

**There is a big difference between water soluble and fat soluble vitamins and minerals**.

**Water soluble vitamins and minerals** are quite safe and these are the ones that you have to replace often if you drink a lot of water.

**Fat soluble vitamins and minerals** get stored in your body fat and do not "wash away" when you drink too much water. You can "overdose" on fat soluble vitamins. They can be toxic.

One or two multivitamin supplements a day will not bring you anywhere near the toxicity levels for fat soluble vitamins, but if you try "mega" doses of vitamins, be sure you understand the recommended dosage amounts for your body size. Talk to you doctor if you are not sure.

Let's use **Vitamin A** (mentioned below) as an example. It is important for skin care.

Vitamin A is a fat soluble vitamin. That means after you eat it, it is absorbed in your upper intestinal tract. About ¼ of what you eat gets into your system. Vitamin A is in many foods as well as supplements.

Strenuous exercise, alcohol, mineral oil, cortisone and some other drugs all interfere with your body's absorption of Vitamin A.

The Recommended Daily Allowances (RDA) for Vitamin A are

> 1,500 IU (International units) for infants
>
> 3,000 IU (International units) for children
>
> 5,000 IU (International units) for adults
>
> Check these often because RDA's change over time.

**Some adults routinely take 10,000 to 25,000 IU of Vitamin A each day to help with acne.**

**Warning: Taking 50,000 IU or more as an adult may be toxic.**

Toxicity symptoms include nausea, vomiting, diarrhea, dry skin, hair loss, headaches, appetite loss, sore lips, and flaky, itchy skin.

If you take a lot of **any** supplement – be smart.  Read about the side effects; **always speak to your doctor before taking more than the RDA**, and watch out for symptoms.

## One study on Vitamin A and Acne

*100 acne patients were given oral does of 100,000 IU of Vitamin A (halibut-liver oil) at bedtime.*

*36 patients were completely relieved of acne, and 43 were relieved except for an occasional pustule. In most cases, responses occurred in less than nine months.*

*(Jon V. Straumfjord, M.D., Astoria, Oregon, reported in Rodale, ed., Prevention, November, 1968.)*

**Vitamin A** is one of the most important vitamins for skin. Vitamin A aids in the growth and repair of body tissues and helps maintain smooth, soft, disease-free skin.

In supplement form, you will get exactly what you need. Too much Vitamin A can cause your skin to become dry and flaky, so it is important to talk to your doctor about the recommended dose for your body size.

The best sources of Vitamin A are from green and orange vegetables (carrots, beet greens, spinach, and broccoli) and milk. In addition to helping your skin, it also helps your vision!

The **B-complex** vitamins, especially riboflavin, pyridoxine, and pantothenic acid, help reduce facial oiliness and blackhead formation.

**Vitamin C** aids in resisting the spread of acne infection.

**Vitamin D** guards

**Omega 3** is also important to good skin health. Omega 3 helps promote healthy skin cells and cell restoration. Your body treats acne like a disease and fights it, which is part of how the scarring occurs.

Having the recommended intake of Omega 3 can help prevent this. Fish oil and salmon are the easiest ways to take this in naturally. If you are a vegetarian, flax seeds (which are great in all types of dishes) and walnuts provide good sources as well.

Just so that we are clear here, even if the supplements do not help directly with your acne, they are promoting better health, which in turn, will help with your acne.

# Acne: A Teenage Nightmare

If you want clear skin, to "look good," and **romance**, you have to give up some of the foods that you love. Period. No debating, no discussion.

> **Teenager's have unique, age related hormonal changes but they also tend to have the worst eating, sleeping, and cleaning habits.**

As you read through this acne book, you will pick up all types of nutritional advice, but **none of it means anything if you do not do the following AT A MINIMUM**.

# TEENAGE "MUST DO" LIST

**<u>Give up soda</u>** (also called pop or tonic). These are sweetened, carbonated beverages like Coke or Pepsi or Mountain Dew. It doesn't matter if they are regular or diet, give them up. Drink lots of water instead. Your skin will clear and look radiant, you'll feel better, and you'll lose weight.

**<u>Give up salty, fried snacks</u>** No potato chips, no nachos, no hot and spicy cheese curls, etc. Nothing. If you "give in" and break this rule, wash your hands and face (using the steps outlined in the blackhead section) immediately afterward each time.

**<u>Give up FRIED fast foods</u>** Sorry, but these are the worst things for your skin (not too great for your health either).

## No FRIED Hamburgers.

## No FRIED Chicken.

## No French FRIES.

## No Fried Fish.

## <u>NOTHING</u> Fried. Get it?

If you "give in" and break this rule (and you will), wash your hands and face (using the steps outlined in the blackhead section) immediately afterward.

## <u>Wash your hands and face</u>

(Use the steps outlined in the blackhead section) each **morning, night, and after every meal at a minimum.**

## Wash after doing ANYTHING that may pass grease, oil, or dirt onto your hands.

You have no idea what sticks to your hands during each meal or after you shake hands or play basketball and then pass to your face unknowing as you scratch and rub. **This is really important**.

## Try not to touch your face

Don't obsess about this but think about it rationally. (This is why it is important to continually wash your hands and face).

*Count how many times each day that you touch your face. How many times? 50? 100? 500? I'm sure it is quite a bit. Now remember that each time you touch your face, you are transferring whatever is on your hands to your face. Did you carry your book?, Put your hands on the seat or table at lunch? Shake hands with someone?, Eat chips? Eat candy, popcorn, or gum? Play baseball, basketball, or football? Sit on the floor or grass?*

*Each time you touch something and then your face you are passing small amounts of what you touched to your face.*

> *My favorite: How many times did you put your hands in your greasy hair and then touch your face?* If you want to keep your face clean, keep your hands off of it.

**Take at least one multi-vitamin/mineral supplement each day**. Your body needs these to repair your skin and if you don't take them, you *will* get acne.

**Put your face in direct sunlight for at least 15-20 minutes each day.** Don't overdo this, twenty minutes is enough. Too much sun can be a bad thing. If you walk to school, sit or play sports outdoors, it is probably enough. If you sit in your room all day, get up, and go outside for a walk.

Sunlight helps your skin in many different ways and aids in the production of Vitamin D.

# Other Alternatives

Changing your diet can be a pain, and I understand that. So, let's say you don't want to change the way you eat. Here are some alternatives.

You don't need to spend tons of money to treat your acne at home.

**You can make your own acne "treatments"** with things you probably already have in your kitchen or bathroom.

**Rubbing alcohol** opens your pores immediately. You do not want to use this more than once a day because it can have the opposite affect and irritate and inflame your skin more than it already is.

A great way to treat acne at home is to make your own **face mask**.

You need oatmeal (plain oatmeal, not the brown sugar flavored oatmeal) and regular yogurt. By regular yogurt, I mean plain yogurt. It is not recommended to make a face mask out of Fruit on the Bottom yogurt. Just buy plain yogurt.

If you have a food processor, it is helpful to grind up the oats, but not necessary. Put the oatmeal in your coffee grinder or lay it out on a paper towel and chop it up. Mix it in with the yogurt until it is pasty. You want the texture to be a little bumpy so that it works as an exfoliate.

Lather it onto your face and let it sit for about fifteen minutes. Wash it off with hot water and soap and rinse off with ice cold water. If your skin is normally extra dry, you can add a little honey to help moisturize while you clean.

If you have to go buy yogurt to do this, buy one of the cheap ones in a small container. You only need two tablespoons of each to make this mask so one small container should last you long enough to make more than one mask.

# Do Not Break The Bank On Expensive Acne Treatments!

**I** may have mentioned earlier you don't need to spend a fortune on acne treatment.

I gave one example of how to make a mask at home with food you probably already have in the kitchen. Most folks have rubbing alcohol in their house already as well.

In addition to those things, you can also use avocado, lemons, oranges, and just about anything else to make a good mask.

**Home treatments save you a fortune.** Even if you need to see a dermatologist, you do not need to spend a fortune. Your insurance probably covers most of the cost. If you do not have insurance, keep working on treatment at home. Like just about everything else, the internet is filled a wide variety of free ways to treat acne at home.

There are some hardcore, super expensive treatments available that will cost you a small fortune and will probably work. Before you try those though, **exhaust every cheap available** option; like changing your diet, changing how you wash your face or the area that is infested, or making homemade washes. **Just because you can do this at home doesn't mean it won't work!**

There are also a ridiculous amount of acne treatments available almost everywhere, including the grocery store, for a relatively low price. **Just because the price is high does not mean it will work better than another product.**

<u>**You have to figure out what is going to work for you and the type of acne you have**</u> - which means you will go through a trial and error process. **You may find certain things actually make your acne worse, which is why I recommend trying only one thing at a time.**

**Avoid those high priced treatments** at stores, online, and even through your dermatologist **until** you have exhausted every option.

The reason is simple, while we know what acne is, we do not know what causes it in you.

Before you drop hundreds of dollars, or before you do that *again*, try eliminating causes first.

# Better Diet Part 3

There will be more than a few references in regard to a **better diet** in this acne book. The reason is simple, if you change everything and continue to eat mass amounts of chocolate and greasy foods; your acne is not going to clear up.

If you are otherwise healthy, maintain a decent diet and exercise, but still eat a bacon cheeseburger every day for lunch; you are not going to get rid of your acne.

Foods that are greasy interfere with your digestion process. The digestion process in delicate and if you are eating foods that irritate that process, your body will not process fats, proteins, and carbohydrates the way is it supposed to.

This in turn, will cause your skin to be greasy, even if only in patches, and the greasy skin, in turn, will produce more acne.

Do you see the connection here? **Bad food is bad for you.** It's a no brainer.

Eat a salad instead of a bacon cheeseburger. Not only is it better for your skin, your heart, and your digestive system, eating a salad for lunch won't leave you feeling like you swallowed a brick and need to take a two hour nap when you get back to work or school.

Good food is important for many reasons, the least of which is your acne.

Every acne treatment in the world will not help you if you do not eat well.

I know fast food tastes good and I know fried food tastes even better. I also know that chocolate is heavenly and dark beer is wonderful. However, most of this stuff is bad for your body and bad for your skin.

It's hard to change your diet in one fell swoop, so **start small.** Eat a salad twice a week for lunch and see if you don't feel better and look better. Keep going until it's a habit instead of a chore and your skin will improve.

**It's not a miracle cure but it is a no-brainer cure.**

# Get Rid Of Oily Skin Naturally

There are many things can contribute to oily skin (diet aside for a minute). As previously noted, hot water, soap, cold water helps get rid of oily skin.

Hot water opens your pores and helps dissolve the oils on your skin. Soap helps dry your skin and remove the funk.

Cold water, as you already know, closes up the pores and follicles again to prevent the funk from finding a new home.

I love **moisturizers**. I like how they make my skin feel and smell. But, **I had to stop using them** because I was trying to get rid of my own oily skin.

Hot water, soap, cold water, **and then talcum powder**. (C'mon, say it with me!) **The talcum powder prevented my skin from getting oilier and doesn't leave a residue like so many moisturizers**.

Talcum powder may leave you feeling like you smell and look like your grandma, but there are vast arrays of powders available that do not smell like grandma.

Another thing to consider is what you put on your face.

Most women wear makeup.

**Most makeup is horrific for your skin. Liquid foundation is horrible for your skin. Most concealer, blushes, and eye shadows are equally bad**.

I understand that you cannot leave your house before putting your face on, I really do. So try to pick makeup that is good for your skin. Read the labels of the makeup you're about to purchase.

**Many makeup companies offer specific makeup for women with acne**. It can include drying agents and even acne medication.

This "acne" makeup tends to be a little pricier, but the cost of cheap makeup is more acne so it is worth it in the long run to fork out a little more cash. Good makeup can help prevent oily skin.

# How Stress Can Cause Acne

Stress can cause or worsen acne. Stress works two ways in causing and worsening acne; it stimulates adrenal glands which then produce more hormones, and it slows the healing process.

Most people tend to eat more or drink more alcohol when they are under stress, stress aids in acne promotion via diet as well.

When we are stressed it affects our health. Stress affects our nervous system. It kicks up our adrenaline (making our skin super oily) and increases our heart rate.

It affects the way we sleep and weakens our immune systems. While these things are bad enough in and of themselves, **stress also makes acne worse**.

If you already have acne, stress makes the flare ups worse because your body is already trying to offset the stress and cannot heal the skin. The skin gets more inflamed than normal.

Stress also causes a form of eczema. Eczema is different from acne but in combination with acne, makes the skin situation even worse.

There are good and bad forms of stress. Getting married or graduating college can be stressful, but these are both generally good stresses. A highly tense work area (think retail management!) or income related stressors are bad stress.

Unfortunately, our body chemistry cannot tell the difference. While mentally you may feel better about getting married than you would about losing your job, your body processes the stress the same way.

It is almost impossible to avoid stress completely, but **it is possible to learn to deal with stress more effectively** and to eliminate stressors in our lives. Some of us have to fight morning traffic and there is nothing we can do about that.

**Learning breathing exercises** that help keep your heart rate normal, help you stay in control and ultimately relieves some stress and your body won't react by making your acne worse.

# Get Rid Of Oily Skin Naturally - Part 2

For a lot of you with acne, your skin is oily, even if only in patches. When your body produces more sweat than necessary or is more oily than necessary, your pores and hair follicles get blocked, causing acne. There are things you can do at home to help fight this, without spending tons of money.

If you remember from an earlier chapter; hot water, soap, ice cold water. It should be a mantra for you by now. If it is not a mantra, say it again with me, "**Hot water, soap, ice cold water**."

This does not cost anything and helps open, cleanse, and close your pores and follicles. Cleaning your face well and often helps oily skin.

**Using soap that dries out your skin can make it worse**, but a good soap can also help, so experiment with soaps. I suggested Zest in an earlier section.

I use it when I break out, but I don't use it otherwise on any other part of my body. It dries my skin really badly and I don't like all the chemicals in it. It's not the only soap out there though, so try different brands. Another good soap is Dove. It is very light on the chemicals, cheap, and smells good.

We already know that stress affects your skin by producing more hormones, making your skin oilier than normal. We know diet has an effect on your skin as well.

**Make sure you don't use oil based makeup or skin creams if your skin is already oily**. Keep drinking lots and lots of water to flush your system and again, hot water, soap, ice cold water.

There is no cure for oily skin so nothing you do will rid you of your skin type. However, there are things like those mentioned above that help offset your oily skin and you can do all this stuff at home at little to no cost.

# Physical Activity Helps Acne

You probably don't want to hear it, but **exercise helps prevent and get rid of acne**. I know, you're wondering how since exercise makes you sweat and sweat makes you oily and your skin is probably already oily. But, it's true and that's what I'm telling you.

Exercise increases your heart rate, blood flow, and oxygen. You get hot and sweaty while exercising and your body releases toxins through your open pores.

**Sweat helps clean dirt, dead skin cells, and other funk from your pores**. Yes, it can also have the opposite effect. (Hot water, soap, ice cold water). So take a shower after you exercise to scrub away sweat and any residue toxins left on your body after a workout.

**Most people drink a lot of water during a workout which helps your body expel toxins. Exercise also lowers stress, enables better sleep, and helps overall body relaxation and all of these things help prevent acne.**

This doesn't mean you have to go join a gym right this second. In fact, you don't need to join a gym at all. Go to your local Dollar Store and buy a jump rope. Jump rope is one of the best exercises you can do. It works your arm and leg muscles, your back and stomach muscles, kicks up your heart rate and is a well rounded cardio exercise. If you don't want to go outside, you can jump rope in your living room. Or jump around your block if you feel like it.

The point is, exercise is good for your body in a lot of ways. **Helping reduce acne is another side effect of exercise.**

Remember though, exercise **will only help with acne prevention and reduction if you wash properly afterwards.**

If you don't wash up when you're through, exercise can actually make your acne worse. So make sure you follow the hot water, soap, and ice cold water practice after each work out session.

# Myths About Acne

Like any type of illness or ailment, people will offer advice on how to fix or cure something and acne is no different. And like most of the advice given to you about most things, you should ignore most of the myths about acne a well.

Chocolate does not cause acne. It can contribute though. If you are eating so much chocolate that you're wondering if it's causing acne, you should probably cut it back. Chocolate does affect your health, and it's not just chocolate, all junk food affects your health negatively.

If you are not eating a balanced, nutritional diet, it is going to affect your skin, have no doubt. By itself though, and on occasion, chocolate should be fine and dark chocolate can actually be beneficial.

Physical activity does not cause acne. As you have already read, it does quite the opposite. Physical activity will help clear up your skin, provided you wash up well when you are done with that activity.

Popping pimples does not get rid of acne.

In fact, **popping any lesions is really bad for your skin**.

The pus that is in acne and pimples is from the dead skin cells, dirt, etc. that has clogged your pores and follicles, it **is essentially an infection**.

**Popping a pimple can make it worse**. While it may remove the surface pus, it is actually pushing the rest of the infection back into the follicle further. This can lead to worse acne that is inflamed and sensitive and can lead to scarring.

**Picking at your skin introduces more dirt to your skin**, which spreads the infection and makes it worse.

Sex does not clear up or cause acne either. Sex is a physical activity like jumping rope (except more fun!). Sex stimulates your brain and your body.

You sweat and secrete toxins just like when you're jumping rope and it is just as important to shower afterwards.

**You want to keep your skin clean and the sweat you produce and rub against during sex needs to be washed off.**

# Acne Pain Relief

Serious acne hurts. The skin becomes inflamed and engorged and it aches and can sometimes even be acute pain. There are different types of acne and severe cases tend to be rooted deep in the skin and can be very painful.

Try **Aspirin**. Of course, ingesting Aspirin or other pain relievers will help. Aspirin though can be used externally as well. If you have ever had a toothache and stuck a piece of Aspirin directly on the tooth and let it dissolve, you know what I am taking about. Some people crush up Aspirin and apply it directly to the outbreak. **Aspirin will reduce the redness and reduce the inflammation**.

**Aloe Vera gel is another do it at home pain relief remedy**. Aloe is naturally soothing and creates a protective barrier that keeps more dirt from getting into your pores. If you have an Aloe plant, break a piece directly off the plant. While it feels greasy going on, it dries quickly and doesn't leave any funky residue.

If you can stand it, put an ice pack onto the spot that is hurting. Ice reduces swelling and the numbing effect may be very beneficial.

You can also try Neosporin. We put it on scrapes and cuts to prevent infection because it is an antibiotic; it works the same way on acne. Talk to your doctor about this and stronger, prescription only versions of Neosporin if you aren't comfortable taking other kinds of pain relief medication.

Of course, again, **the best pain treatment is prevention**.

Remember, "Hot water, soap, ice cold water." If the pain is so severe that none of the at-home-over-the-counter pain relief suggestions work, you really should go see a dermatologist who can prescribe you something stronger if you need it.

# Acne Scars

Before even considering whether to think about treatment for your acne scars, you need to be acne free. The reason for this is obvious. If you are still battling with acne and treat current scars, you will have to treat new scars at another time. If you're not cleared up yet, scar treatment won't work.

The most important thing to consider when looking into acne scar treatment is to be realistic in your expectation. **Not all scars are created equal** and the types of scars will affect the way treatment is done and the level of success.

One of the most well known and popular treatments is **collagen injections**. Collagen injections work by filling out the scars and making them less noticeable. The upside is it generally works and with makeup, your scars may not be noticeable at all. The downside is collagen injections are expensive, insurance doesn't usually pay for them and the process has to be repeated every four months.

**Laser treatment** is another option available. This type of surgery alters the scar tissue and removes redness. Laser treatment is a good option for lighter, less severe scars, but this too may take more than one visit and can be painful.

**Dermabrasion** is another well known acne scar treatment. It works by using a high-speed brush to remove the surface skin layer and changes the contour of the scars. If they are on surface, superficial scars may be removed altogether. Deeper scars will lose their depth. This too may take more than one treatment and it's success is dependent upon the type of scars you have.

**A** treatment that is not new, but not very well known is **Autologous fat transfer**. This works in a way similar to collagen except it is using fat from another part of your body. The fat is injected just beneath the surface of your skin to elevate deep scars. It works well because your body recognizes your fat (no rejection).

The downside to this treatment is it needs to be done more than once, about once a year because your body will reabsorb the fat.

# Back Acne

**Back acne** is caused the same way facial acne is. However, back acne can actually be harder to get rid of. It's harder to wash your back, for starters.

**Buy a body scrubber**. Most grocery stores carry them and they don't cost a lot of money.

**Hot water, soap, ice cold water- just like your face**. While you can stop wearing makeup and change things up to prevent introducing new bacteria to your face, it is much harder to do with your back.

**I**f you are in school - junior high, high school, or college - you probably carry around a **backpack**. Those straps are rubbing against your shoulders and back the whole time you have the backpack on. This not only irritates your skin, but it keeps the pores open through stimulation and it keeps the area sweaty and oily.

If you can, get a pack with wheels and drag it around with you. If it's not possible, make sure you give your shoulders and back plenty of time to air out at home.

**Wear looser fitting, always clean clothes** as well. I know the style is form fitting shirts. Shirts that are tight don't allow your skin to breathe when you sweat and work against your skin the same way backpacks do.

**B**ack acne is not usually the same type of acne that is on your face and while it can be severe and difficult to get rid of, **keeping your back dry and clean clears it up faster than facial acne**.

Try swimming. I know that if you have back acne the last thing you want to do is put on a bathing suit so the whole world can see the acne on your body. However, the chemicals used to treat swimming pools tend to dry out your skin and will help clear up your back acne quickly.

# Do Not Touch Your Acne!

**I** may only write about this ten more times in this acne book because it is so important.

Acne starts with clogged hair follicles (pores). It is not clear why some people's follicles get blocked and others do not, although genes can come into play.

If one of your parents had acne, chances are you will too. Once the follicles are blocked by dirt, the oil that normally comes through your skin as sweat can't get out and bacteria starts to grow where the oil is.

Blackheads and whiteheads are considered acne, they are just not inflamed. Whiteheads and blackheads can release the oil and pus and heal. However, the follicle wall can rupture.

**The rupture of the follicle wall causes inflammatory acne.** The rupture itself is caused by people with acne picking at their faces or trying to pop the whiteheads and blackheads. The pressure of trying to pop the pimples can cause the follicle walls to rupture.

> **Aside from turning blackheads and whiteheads into inflamed, red, painful acne, touching your face introduces new dirt and bacteria to your face and makes the current condition worse.**

Like your mother probably told you, keep your hands away from your face. If you must touch your face, if you put in contact lenses, apply makeup with your fingers, or just need to scratch an itch, make sure you wash your hands with antibacterial soap before you touch your face.

**The goal, of course, is to not touch your face at all, but that is pretty impractical. At the very least, make sure your hands and fingers are clean.**

Aside from the obvious of not picking at your skin or popping your acne, **there are a lot of dirty, bacterial covered items that come in contact with your face on a regular basis**.

While you may not pick at your face, you probably **rest your chin or cheek on your hand** at some point and you probably don't wash your hands. Be aware of that.

**The phone you use at home and at work is covered in germs and dirt, so is your cell phone.**

You can't stop using the phone, but you can clean it beforehand or wash your face afterwards.

# Use A Gentle Face Wash

Exfoliates are great for our skin. Our skin feels refreshed after scrubbing with the homemade or store bought exfoliates and we generally feel really clean afterwards. The problem with harsh exfoliates when you have acne is they can irritate and inflame skin that is already irritated and inflamed.

Rather than using a harsh exfoliate, use something gentle (hot water, soap, ice cold water) that will be easy on your skin. While you want to get your face clean **it is super important to not irritate it** beyond what it already is.

Oatmeal is a gentle exfoliate and you probably already have some at home, mix oatmeal and yogurt (see the chapter on how to make homemade face masks) and use that in addition to soap and water to help your face get clean without irritating it.

Another great exfoliate product you can use that is really gently is **Dove Gentle Exfoliate**. The reason why I like Dove so much in general is there are not a lot of chemicals in their products. Even some of the best products have a lot of chemicals and even if the product is billed as being gentle on the skin, the chemicals can irritate your skin even more.

Dove products seem to me to be less harsh and have fewer chemicals than other brands. Their gentle exfoliate cleans well without leaving behind a residue and without irritation. **Like choosing the soap you will use as part of your daily cleaning, you may want to try different brands and see which one works best for you**.

Know that the Dove product comes highly recommended on most acne sites though. It is gentle and because of that does not irritate the skin like other cleaners do.  Regardless of the type of cleaner you use, **it is important for you to wash gently rather than scrub**. Even the gentlest of cleaners can irritate your skin if you are scrubbing rather than lightly washing.

# Get A Good Moisturizer

Moisturizers are oily by nature. They are used to replace oil that gets blocked by acne and should be soothing and leave a protective film over the skin. Because most people with acne use a variety of products that treat and dry the acne covered skin, moisturizers are important to help maintain balance on the skin. Moisturizers help keep the oils and water in the skins that are needed for healthy skin.

The best, most gentle facial cleansers can still leave your skin dry and flaky, especially the skin around your acne. **While drying out oily skin is helpful, you do not want to completely dry out the area or the area surrounding the break outs**.

A good moisturizer is important to healthy skin care. With acne, **you do not want a moisturizer that is oily**. I love Oil of Olay products, but I can only use them on my hands, feet, and elbows. Anywhere else and I break out really badly because of the excess oil in them. (It could be dependent upon the specific type I am using though).

It is important when choosing a moisturizer to find one that is oil free but that still promotes **hydration**. Check the labels of what you are going to purchase. Somewhere on the bottle it should say, "noncomedogenic." **This means that the moisturizer is designed to not clog your pores**, which is important when combating acne.

The best moisturizers for acne have three things in common:
1. They will help protect the skin against new acne outbreaks.
2. They can treat acne, help prevent scarring and further inflammation
3. They help balance the skin's natural oils and help keep your pores from becoming blocked.

# Be Careful Of Your Makeup

**There is makeup that is not only acne friendly, but skin friendly in general**. Makeup, especially cheap makeup can make acne worse by plugging your pores with chemicals that are bad for the skin. Women know makeup can get expensive, but there are reasonably priced brands available.

Look for makeup that is **water based**. If you are treating your face already with acne medication and moisturizer, you will want to wear makeup that is as gentle and chemical free as possible.

**Water based makeup tends to be better on the skin**. There are also **foundations available that have acne medicine in them** that don't smell horrible and look good on the skin.

**In addition to using water based, acne medicated foundation; you will want foundation with SPF in it as well**. You are killing three birds with one stone this way. Your face will be protected from the sun, from dirt and other gunk that can clog your pores, and you will be treating your acne at the same time.

Matte foundations dry into a powder-type finish and leave the skin smooth. Using this type of foundation allows you to wear one less type of makeup.

Aside from foundation, there are **eye shadows, blushes, and lipsticks** all designed to help prevent acne breakouts. If your skin is very oily, use powder eye shadow and powder blushes rather than the crème one.

**The cream shadows and blushes are usually oil based and even with a good foundation or concealer, those oily products is going to get into your pores**.

It is important to **wash your face well before putting on makeup and to wash your face well when you remove makeup**.

Even forgetting to wash makeup off one time can cause acne break outs. (I sound like a skipping record, I know, but use the hot water, soap, and cold water treatment to get rid of your makeup).

# Acne Products

I will not endorse any "name brand" acne prevention products here as, quite frankly, I believe you can solve your problem without them and do so naturally. I will mention one "ingredient" that are widely available from many companies.

**Benzoyl Peroxide** has been used for a long time to treat acne. It acts as a peeling agent, clearing pores and encouraging skin turn over. This lowers the amount of bacteria that can live on your skin and benzoyl peroxide works as an antibacterial agent also.

The bacteria that clogs your pores and causes acne cannot live in an environment that is full of oxygen. There are different levels of benzoyl peroxide you can use in creams from 2.5% to 10%.

The scientific research done on benzoyl peroxide use for acne treatment says the lowest percent is just as effective as the highest percent. The lower percentage is less likely to irritate your skin.

In starting with the lower percentage dose, start application twice a day. If it does not seem to be helping, and does not irritate your skin, up the amount of times you apply. If you are using it up to five times a day and it's not helping, then go for a higher percentage.

Before each application it is important to wash your face and hands and let them completely dry before putting the cream or ointment on. Pat your face dry with a towel and wait an additional few minutes to make sure your face is all the way dry.

Even the lowest dose can irritate your skin, but it is recommended you use it for at least a week before giving up. Once your skin adjusts to it, the irritation will lessen. Benzoyl Peroxide is also notorious for causing dry, flaky skin, so it is important to have a good non-irritating moisturizer on hand as well.

# Mild to Moderate Acne

There are two different variants of acne: **mild to moderate and severe**.

**M**ild to moderate acne is easier to treat and deal with than the severe types. Mild to moderate acne is referred to as Acne Vulgaris and includes blackheads, whiteheads, papules, pustules.

**Whiteheads** happen when the pore is completely blocked. The blockage traps oils, bacteria and dead skin cells and makes the surface of the acne white.

These usually do not last as long as other types of acne but before you start popping them (read the other sections to see why popping pimples and acne is actually bad for your skin).

**Blackheads** happen when the pore is only partially blocked. The partial blockage allows some of the oils, bacteria and dead skin cells to drain to the surface and spread, causing more blackheads or whiteheads.

Dirt itself is not bad for your skin, and the color of the blackhead is not due to dirt. It is the skin pigment reacting to the oxygen in the air. These are almost impossible to pop and should not be popped either.

**Papules are blackheads that are inflamed**. The inflammation blocks the head and a true papule will not have a visible head on it. The papules are also red and very tender. Trying to pop these will increase the likelihood of scarring and does not do any good.

**Pustules are whiteheads that are inflamed**. Usually the outside of pustule is red and has a white or yellow center. The center is infection caused by the trapped oil, dead skin, and bacteria.

Even though you want to, it is very important to not pop any of the acne on your face or elsewhere. Popping leads to scarring and spreading the infection from the acne across your face to other areas. The dirt and bacteria on your hands can also make the infection worse.

# Severe Acne

There are a few types of acne which are worse than the mild to moderate variety: **nodules and cyst**s. They are both generally painful and usually require a trip to the dermatologist. Severe acne is not that common. Of the severe type, there are four categories.

**Acne conglobata** is the most severe form of acne vulgaris. It tends to be more common in males than females. They are large lesions that are connected and the sufferer usually has an inordinately large amount of blackheads also.

They usually show up on the face, chest, back, butt, upper arms, and thighs. This type of acne usually lasts for years and is difficult to treat because it is often resistant to common treatments. The treatment requires trips to a dermatologist and very aggressive, consistent, longterm treatment.

**Pyoderma Faciale** is severe acne that affects females. This form of acne is large, painful nodules, pustules, and sores that can leave severe scarring. It starts quickly and can occur in women who have never had so much as a breakout. If treated correctly, it generally does not last longer than a year but if not treated immediately will leave severe scarring. Aggressive treatment can usually clear it up in a year.

**Acne Fulminans** generally affects younger men and is extremely severe. The onset of this type of acne is usually abrupt and is evident in the ulcer-like appearance. Scarring is so severe with this type of acne that is often referred to as disfiguring. Fever and joint aches also accompany this type of acne and it does not respond to antibiotics. When a person has this type of acne, oral steroids are generally the only treatment that works.

**Gram-Negative Folliculitis** is an acne vulgaris complication. It is very rare and looks like regular acne as it forms pustules and cysts. It is thought that this complication occurs as a result of longterm treatment for acne vulgaris.

# How To Cut Back Stress To Help With Acne

Because stress stimulates hormone production and weakens the immune system, if you are already acne prone or suffering from acne, stress can make it worse. We can't eliminate stress from our lives entirely, but here are a **few exercises** that can help you cope with stress when it happens.

Coping with stress can help lessen stress and that will prevent your body from excess hormone production.

**Breathe**. Of course we all breathe all the time and don't even think about. **Slow deep breathing exercises** help calm the mind and body and are something that can be done anywhere. While sitting in traffic is not the ideal place for meditation, you can use deep breathing exercises in traffic, in the office, or at home.

The best position is to sit cross legged with your back straight. Keep the tip of your tongue on the edge of your upper teeth.

Exhale completely through your mouth and count to four. While exhaling, pull your stomach in. This helps get all the air out of your diaphragm. Now close your mouth and inhale through your nose, pushing your stomach out and count to four in your head.

Hold your breath and count to seven.

Exhale through your mouth again, pulling in your stomach and count to eight. The eight count marks one breath. Do this again three more times.

The counting and the exact numbers are important to make sure the breaths are complete. **This helps calm you mentally and physically**. Of course, you want to be alert when you are driving, but even the best of us get stressed out in traffic and practicing a shorter version of this breathing exercise can help calm nerves in traffic.

Breathing exercises will not cure acne, obviously. But learning to cope with stress as it happens does help your body remain healthy and this in turn helps your acne.

# Natural Acne Treatments

There are a lot of natural ways to treat acne and I think it best to break those up into two sections so I can be a little more detailed.

The list here, and in the second section are things that have been touched on in other sections. These are less common ways to treat acne naturally. With the exception of extreme acne, these natural treatments do help clear the skin up and are much more cost effective in comparison to over the counter medications.

**Aloe Vera plant**: Aloe has been used for a long time medicinally. It helps restore skin after burns and wounds and acts as an anti-inflammatory and immunity booster.

In addition to being helpful with these things, if you are fortunate enough to have an aloe plant, you can pick a piece directly from the plant, cut it open and apply directly to the skin. It has a soothing effect as well.

Heat can also be used to help with acne. Heat kills bacteria and will aid in the healing of an infected area. There are products you can buy designed specifically to heat and treat acne.

They work almost like mini blow dryers and are used a pimple at a time for a minute each and while it can be time consuming, it is a painless way to treat acne at home. The heat can dry your skin, so following a heat treatment with aloe would be a good way to go.

Earlier Aspirin was mentioned as a topic treatment for acne pain reduction. Naproxen and ibuprofen can be used the same way.

Crush the pill up and apply it directly to the acne. All three help with pain and Naproxen and ibuprofen are also anti-inflammatory. Once the pain has lessoned and your acne is no longer swollen so bad, other treatments can be used without causing pain and irritation.

**Vitamin B3** is a good way to help treat acne naturally. B3 in gel form can be used as a topical antibiotic and can be taken as a supplement. B3 is a natural anti-inflammatory and helps your body produce more collagen and keratins, helping your skin heal better.

It is available through prescription or at any pharmacy, health store, or grocery store. Just pop open the gel cap and put the gel directly on to the acne site.

**Tea Tree Oil** is another natural remedy that is readily available just about anywhere. You'll need the 5% strength for it to be effective and it works the same way benzoyl peroxide does except it doesn't dry your skin as much. It can have an irritating effect initially, but works as an anti-inflammatory and the irritation shouldn't last very long.

Zinc taken orally also helps with inflammation of acne. Like any vitamin, too much zinc is bad for you and hard for your body to digest without the proper intake of food so it's important if you start taking a zinc supplement to take it with food and start with a lower dosage. 15 mg is the RDA and many acne suffers increase that to 25 mg to be the most effective.

There are many ways to treat acne naturally and many ways to help prevent acne from returning once it's gone. Natural methods are a good way to go if you are trying to maintain a healthier lifestyle. Because natural remedies are becoming more popular, it is easier to find these things and easier to find information about what might work best for you.

**All of the natural remedies listed here can easily be found at a health food store, pharmacy, or grocery store in the vitamin section.**

# When To See A Dermatologist

Most people breakout at some point in their lives. Even one or two pimples can feel like a major breakout when we are young or if the pimples are huge, red, and irritated.

A lot of people do not go to the doctor to get treated for acne because it can get expensive and they are just pimples right? A lot of us believe that the acne will go away as we get older and a lot of times it does.

But for those who have never had a problem with acne and have an outbreak in adulthood or for those teenagers who cannot function socially because of their acne, a dermatologist may be the way to go and the sooner the better.

Most people won't go to a dermatologist if their acne is mild and I don't blame them. When considering whether or not to go to a dermatologist, ask yourself the following questions:

- Do you have painful nodules, blackheads and whiteheads, and red spots on your skin?
- Do you have scars or the beginnings of scars where your acne has cleared up?
- Are you embarrassed by your acne?
- Does your acne make you shy around new people?
- Do you have dark skin and darker spots where the acne has cleared?
- Does your acne make you depressed?

The guideline is if you answer yes to any of those questions you should see a dermatologist. If you feel your lifestyle is inhibited by your acne, **and you cannot clear it up on your own**, then go see a dermatologist.

If you have moderate acne or severe acne it can be difficult to clear up on your own and if you have been unable to do so, then yes, go see a dermatologist.

**I** even recommend a dermatologist visit for an initial consultation. It gives you an idea of the severity of your acne, looks for other problems, and can give you peace of mind. Remember though, **their business is treating skin disorders so you are not just a patient, but also a source of income to them.**

# Acne and Self Esteem

Even as adults, acne sufferers can have self esteem problems. Most people rebound fairly quickly if they are able to clear up their acne in a short amount of time, but when it acne is a long term battle, it can lead to self esteem problems and depression.

If you are doing everything you can to battle acne or if you have clear skin but scarring from previous acne and it affects your self esteem, you should talk to your doctor or dermatologist about a recommendation for a therapist who deals specifically with self esteem issues.

Being able to talk about things often helps and being able to find ways to offset or change how you feel about yourself helps even more.

If you are fortunate and made it through acne with no scarring, you may still have self esteem issues. Even acne that does not leave scars can be disfiguring while it's there.

It is hard to imagine yourself at the prom or party when your face and back are covered in acne. It is hard to imagine yourself leading a meeting or teleconference with clients when you are battling acne. Event small events like meeting your kid's teacher for the first time can be difficult to face if you are battling acne.

There is nothing wrong with getting counseling. Our self esteem affects our mental state and when we have low self esteem, we usually are depressed or headed that way. People who are depressed have lower immune systems and tend to eat poorly and both of those contribute to acne flare ups.

Getting rid of acne is not only a physical issue; it is a mental one as well. If we are mentally healthy, it is easier to stay physically healthy. So before you give up or even start to feel like giving up, talk to your doctor.

# Adult Acne

You have negotiated the teenage years with relatively minor damage. After a long battle with teenage acne you have beaten it and moved on with your life only to wake up one morning at 35 to see the tell-tale signs of acne staring back at you in the mirror.

What happened? You probably thought only teenagers get acne or adults with bad hygiene.

**Adult acne** affects 25% of men and 50% of women at some point during adulthood. Keep in mind though, most everyone gets a few pimples here and there and the statistics above are not for a few pimples, it is for breakouts of acne and that is different. Ultimately, age doesn't matter when it comes to acne; it can happen at any time.

Welcome to the horrible world of adult acne. Just when you thought it was over, it crops back up and you have to deal with it again. The good news is as an adult you are better equipped emotionally, mentally, physically, and monetarily to deal with acne. The quickest, most obvious way to deal with adult acne is to go to the doctor.

If you do not want to go to the doctor or if you are embarrassed about getting treated for adult acne, there are a lot of over the counter medicines you can buy or home remedies you can try to get rid of it effectively.

Topical treatments may help with your acne quickly. Oatmeal and honey treatments at home can be effective as well. If you have tried everything you can think of then it is time to put your embarrassment aside and head to the doctor.

Adult acne doesn't need to be a source of embarrassment and it should not rule your life.

# Do Not Spend A Lot Of Money On Acne Treatments!

Because acne can come and go, you do not want to spend a lot of money on treatments. Even over the counter medications can get expensive if you are not careful about what you buy. If you have insurance, go the doctor. It may be the cheaper option in the long run if you need long-term or constant treatment for acne because your insurance pays for most of it, including prescriptions.

If you do not want to go to the doctor or you do not have insurance, or if you just don't have the time to make an appointment and go, there are **other low cost options available**.

Most drugstore and grocery stores have a **store brand version** of just about everything. If you know a specific type of acne product you want to use, **check the active ingredients and the amount of the ingredient in that product**.

Check the store brand label and see if the ingredients match. Probably they do. If they do, **buy the store brand**. Generally store brands run anywhere from a few dollars to five or ten dollars cheaper than name brands. If the active ingredient is the same, it is essentially the same product in a not as fancy box.

In the same regard, **look for coupons or manufacture's rebates**. A lot of acne treatment products offer rebates or have money back offers for purchasing their products. This is a great way to get a name brand product for a cheaper price.

If you are all about do-it-yourself options, there are a lot of things you can use at home to help with your acne that are inexpensive or free. If you have **aloe plants** in your yard, use those to help with your acne. You probably already have **Aspirin** in your home that can be used as well.

Read this acne book and re-read this acne book.

# Oral Antibiotic And Retinoid Acne Treatment

Because acne is essentially an infection caused from the oil in blocked pores, **antibiotics** can effectively treat many types of acne. Some are one a day, some are multiple times a day pills.

While antibiotics help kill the bacteria in the infection, they do not reduce oil secretion which is usually the initial cause of the blocked pores. Antibiotics are becoming less common in treating acne though because the bacteria that causes acne is becoming resistant.

And while antibiotics will clear up acne, there will be further flare ups within a few days of stopping treatment if a topic treatment is not used in addition to the oral antibiotics.

That is not to say one shouldn't consider using oral antibiotics. One type of antibiotic, **minocycline**, has been found in sub-antimicrobial doses to improve acne. It also has anti-inflammatory effects which helps prevent new flare ups.

Because the dose is so low, it does not kill the bacteria that causes acne and won't induce resistance. This may be an option if you have taken antibiotics before and your acne has become immune to that treatment.

**Oral retinoid** is another option that works for the longer term in complete removal or extreme reduction of acne. It cleared and improved acne in 80% of the patients who have used it. It can have side effects and most doctors or dermatologists who prescribe it only do so as a last resort if all else has failed. The drug also causes severe birth defects and doctors require women who are taking it to use two separate types of birth control while under treatment. Personally, I would avoid this if possible.

Before deciding this is the first course of action you want to take in treating acne, it is important to talk to your doctor at length. Both of these options can have severe side effects and are only recommended after all else fails.

# One Of My Favorites

**I** have to be honest; I personally like the Clinique brand. I do not actually use anything by that company on a regular basis, but my grandmother was a big fan and the packaging and smells of Clinique remind me of her.

I know that is not a good reason to recommend or not recommend a product, but I can't help myself.

**Clinique Acne Solutions Emergency Gel Lotion works**

The gel lotion works, not because it is a Clinique product, but because it is a benzoyl peroxide based product. As mentioned earlier, benzoyl peroxide helps remove pimples.

The gel lotion also unclogs pores, eliminates redness, and helps balance out oil production.

Clinique is not a cheap brand especially if you need to treat your acne regularly; it is however, a good brand and this product works well for me.

# General Information With Regard To Acne

There are many reasons to be healthy, the least of which is your acne. However, your overall health can affect the level of acne.

**A diet high in fruits and vegetables** is beneficial for your overall health and helps with acne.

**A good balanced diet** keeps your immune system healthy enabling it to fight bacteria that causes acne. A balanced diet also helps how your body processes and eliminates toxins which also help your body fight acne.

Acne can be from allergic reactions and eliminating certain foods while adding others foods to your diet may be a way to figure out if you are allergic to a certain food.

**Exercise** is beneficial as well, increasing your heart rate and helping your body sweat out toxins.

Because acne is caused by bacteria, **good hygiene** is important too. Acne affects all types of people and is indiscriminate, so just because you have acne does not mean you are not hygienic, but it can mean you need to be more aware of **proper face washing techniques**.

**Stress** affects your immune system and your mental health and both of those have affects on your body's ability to fight off acne.

There are a lot of small changes you can make in all areas of your life that will improve your overall health and therefore improve your acne.

Another thing to consider is **how often you wash your sheets and pillow cases**. Dust is essentially dead skin cells and they accumulate everywhere. If you wash your sheets and pillow cases once a week, you may want to try washing them every other day to see if that helps.

Cut your caffeine intake as well. This helps not only with acne, but with stress and overall health as well. If your caffeine intake is high, cut back some each day.

# The Last Word On Acne

**Thanks again** for purchasing this natural acne treatment book.

I've really tried to include everything that I know about acne causes and cures in here.

**Don't give up.** The only way that you won't solve your acne problem is if you stop and give up. Keep trying everything in this acne book.

Everyone is different. Each skin type is slightly different and each type of acne is slightly different. The right treatment is going to be different for each person. Creams and ointments may work great for me. You may find that just washing your face, hands, and hair more often works for you.

## Improvements in hygiene, vitamins, proper diet and rest should work for 75% of you.

Before beginning treatment of any type, you really should talk to a doctor first. A doctor can guide and help you choose the treatment that will work best for you and can also give you recommendations for dermatologists if he or she feels you need one.

Acne can be a crippling infection to battle emotionally and if you are feeling down or losing self esteem for it, it is important to seek professional help. Again, your doctor can recommend someone for you.

The number of over the counter and do it yourself treatments are unlimited. There is an option for everyone that will effectively treat acne. **The trick is in finding what is right for you** and it can get discouraging if you have been dealing with it for years.

**Keep trying** though, not only individual treatments but more than one at a time. Treatments that offer more methods in one dose usually work because it is attacking your acne in different ways at the same time.

Ultimately, the treatment you seek and use is **up to you**. Just know that there are **plenty of options available** and there is something that **will** work for you.

www.ingramcontent.com/pod-product-compliance
Lightning Source LLC
Chambersburg PA
CBHW070121010626
45794CB00012B/1031